Anti-Inflammation Diet

The Complete Guide to Living Pain and Drug Free-
includes a 14 day meal plan and delicious recipes for
success

By Caroline G.Hawley

Text Copyright © Caroline G. Hawley

Legal & Disclaimer

Legal & Disclaimer

The information contained in this book is not designed to replace or take the place of any form of medicine or professional medical advice. The information in this book has been provided for educational and entertainment purposes only.

The information contained in this book has been compiled from sources deemed reliable, and it is accurate to the best of the Author's knowledge; however, the Author cannot guarantee its accuracy and validity and cannot be held liable for any errors or omissions. Changes are periodically made to this book. You must consult your doctor or get professional medical advice before using any of the suggested remedies, techniques, or information in this book.

Upon using the information contained in this book, you agree to hold harmless the Author from and against any damages, costs, and expenses, including any legal fees potentially resulting from the application of any of the information provided by this guide. This disclaimer applies to any damages or injury caused by the use and application, whether directly or indirectly, of any advice or information presented, whether for breach of contract, tort, negligence, personal injury, criminal intent, or under any other cause of action.

You agree to accept all risks of using the information presented inside this book. You need to consult a professional medical practitioner in order to ensure you are both able and healthy enough to participate in this program.

Table of Contents

Dedication

"It is more important to know what sort of a person has a disease than to know what sort of disease a person has."

Hippocrates

To patients with chronic inflammatory conditions- whose suffering is often side-lined or underestimated by society, and to those who don't know where to turn for help- This book has been especially written with you in mind!

Introduction

Case History -Explosive joint pains

"I get these terrible, terrible pains in my joints. They start out as mild spasms but can get much worse over time. I've also noticed that I have tender, warm and swollen joints. I can even feel small bumps on my armpits. They appear to be like tiny lumps of tissue and are worrying me sick- to the point that it's affecting my daily life. You see, there are times when I feel so stiff that it becomes difficult to wake up. In fact sometimes, the pain becomes so severe that it leads to fever.

There must be something terribly wrong with me because these symptoms have progressively become more visible lately. Yet, there are times when I feel absolutely ok and have no pain at all- none whatsoever. I believe I'm not somatising things- well, I certainly hope I'm not. So what the matter with me and why do I go through these bouts of pain ever so frequently? Is there something to be worried about? The status of "not knowing" is pushing my anxiety to the limit and not helping at all!"

If this sounds even remotely close to what you're going through, then read on, for you might be experiencing hallmark symptoms of rheumatoid arthritis and the first tell-tale signs of chronic inflammation. You see, in most cases, inflammation is "normal" and is your immune's response to injury or damage. While the symptoms range from pain, swelling, redness and warmth, they are mostly normal and are signs that tell you your body is healing well. Now occasionally, these symptoms can last for a bit longer, sometimes even lasting for a few days. This too is quite normal and is possibly your body's immune system responding to conditions such as injury or infection.

However, if the symptoms last longer than usual and become persistent enough to be noticed, then there's a likelihood that things might have gone south and you might be suffering with chronic inflammation. Simply put, chronic inflammation is when your body loses its ability to supress the inflammatory responses and in the process, begins damaging healthy tissues and causing itself more harm. Known to affect people across all cultures, the condition can damage your intestinal lining and cause gastrointestinal problems, heart ailments and rheumatoid arthritis. Unfortunately, this, is listing only a few of the host of conditions chronic inflammation is known to influence.

Understanding the condition while recognising your symptoms for what they're worth is the first step towards addressing and even overcoming the difficulty. Choosing the right diet is the next all-important step and can make a positive difference in easing your symptoms.

Thankfully, this is exactly what I've set out to achieve in this book. While I admit right here, at the very beginning of this book, that I cannot cure the condition of chronic inflammation, I promise to leave you with powerful tools (dietary tips and recipes in specific) that help overcome any painful symptoms to achieve long-lasting health. In these pages, I share with you my expert knowledge in the field of nutrition and suggest dietary changes to help fight inflammation and prevent it from getting worse. Most importantly, I hope to address any plaguing questions that you might have on the condition while positively influencing the lives of those suffering from the illness, both psychologically and physiologically. In this book, you'll find ways to:

- Become aware of your symptoms
- Embrace dietary and lifestyle changes to take control of it
- Reduce, avoid or eliminate foods that are known to aggravate your discomfort

- Embrace healthy and proven diets that help you stay healthy and symptom-free

- Lead a healthy, vibrant and full-filling life

Well, that's not all- I also leave you with 45 lip-smacking recipes that make eating healthy- EASY!

On that note, I warmly welcome you to my book titled, "Anti-Inflammation Diet" and encourage you to soak into all that is presented in it. As always, I've made this a practical guide, giving you dietary and lifestyle tips for a healthy life. I urge you take a moment to try out the guidelines even as you read the book. I guarantee that you'll be pleasantly surprised at the positive difference it is going to make.

Stay blessed,

Caroline

Inflammation-The enemy INSIDE You

Picture your body as a fortress built for endurance and long-lasting health. It's also built to defend itself from pathogens. While your skin and mucus membranes act as its first line of defence, enzymes such as Lysozyme that are found in sweat and tears help destroy any potential invaders chemically. However, despite these significant barriers, occasionally, pathogens can find their way into your body and into your bloodstream, causing damage and infection as they feed on the other good organisms that house inside.

Upon infection, your body switches its defence mechanism and triggers an inflammatory response that alerts the immune system of an infection. This response, in turn, alerts white blood and protein cells to repair the injury, triggering a slow burning sensation that usually shows up in the form of redness, swelling or pus. Well, this process, however complicated it might seem, is absolutely normal and is a sign of a healthy and functional immune system.

Inflammation: Acute or Chronic?

Now occasionally, when the injury or illness gets deeper and hence requires a longer healing period, the inflammatory response can linger for a little longer; sometimes, even lasting for a period of few days. This type of inflammation is a direct consequence of an injury and is called acute inflammation. If you've ever been bruised or injured, you've most likely witnessed this in action too. So what you probably recognized as the injury itself was in essence, your body's response to injury or damage repair. The tender, throbbing and uncomfortable hotspots that you felt were all part of the healing process. This too is quite normal and is your body's response to the injury or illness. Some hallmark cases that lead to acute inflammation are:

- Injuries such as a sprained ankle or a broken arm
- Bacterial or viral infections
- Sunstrokes
- Deep Incisions

When inflammation lingers long after the job is done or malfunctions in anyway, what was once your best friend can quickly become your worst enemy, leading to a prolonged symptom called chronic inflammation. When inflammation becomes chronic, your body's natural defence system begins to malfunction in ways that are destructive. Not only does it influence the inflammation to linger longer but it can also attack your joints, tissues and blood vessels, creating havoc in areas that were once healthy and pain-free. It is only then that the slow burning throb you once thought was "normal" becomes a five-alarm fire.

So, is it something to be worried about?

You see, as discussed before, having an inflammatory response is "normal" and is your immune system's natural and healthy response to cellular damage. However, believing that it's normal for it to persist for no apparent reason is wrong. While chronic inflammation cannot be the root cause of any disease, it can be the first tell-tale symptom of certain chronic and even life-threatening diseases.

For years, researchers have linked chronic inflammation to rheumatoid arthritis, multiple sclerosis, and asthma. If that was not enough, with the advancement in medicine today, researchers fear that the buck doesn't stop there. In addition to the above problems, chronic inflammation, if undetected and not treated can trigger the onset of life-threatening diseases such heart attack, strokes, diabetes, Alzheimer's and even cancer.

Signs and symptoms of chronic inflammation

Most often, the red flag for chronic inflammation only shows up when a disease associated with it is either left undetected or untreated and hence has become prominent enough to make its presence felt. Some diseases that are commonly linked to chronic inflammation are heart ailments, cancer, rheumatoid arthritis and a blanket of autoimmune diseases including Ulcerative Colitis and Crohn's disease.

Some of the signs include:

- Perennial pain (usually in the joints and muscles)
- Allergies such as asthma (especially if the condition is in its most aggressive state)
- Hyper tension
- Increased levels of sugar
- Intestinal ulcers
- Irritable bowel syndrome (IBS)
- Exhaustion
- Skin breakouts

When and how do I test for chronic inflammation?

If you've been experiencing any of the above problems for a substantial period of time, then it's time you get yourself tested for chronic inflammation. Now, while there isn't a single bullet test that can ascertain chronic inflammation, there are a series of tests that when diagnosed along with your symptoms, can help reveal the levels of inflammation in your body.

The most common markers used to detect chronic inflammation are:

- High levels of C-Reactive Protein, indicating an infection in the body
- Elevated levels of Homocysteine
- High levels of Ferritin in the blood
- High levels of HDL cholesterol
- High levels of Monocyte, also considered to be a consequence of chronic inflammation
- High levels of Glucose in the blood

Now, if the combination of these tests indicate that you have signs of chronic inflammation, then it's imperative that you focus on making anti-inflammatory choices from here on.

Causal Factors

Identifying trigger elements

Infection and injury

Infection and injury are among the first causes of inflammation. The moment your body senses an infection or injury, it sends out signals to the immune system to repair the affected area. Just as white blood and protein cells attend to the affected area, they trigger inflammation all around it.

Stress and anxiety

Many people find that elevated levels of stress or anxiety triggers an overactive inflammatory response. Some others have witnessed a change in lifestyle to trigger the symptoms. Whether it is something as regular as starting work and leaving home or something more life-changing as getting married or having a baby, if you're stressed about something, you're also more likely to trigger signals that cause inflammation.

Obesity

It makes sense that when you pile on extra weight (especially when you do so suddenly); your fat cells too begin to bulge. Not knowing if the bulge is due to fat or an impending problem, your immune system triggers signals to the white blood cells to repair the bulge. This causes inflammation which in turn can make healthy cells resistant to insulin. Given that insulin is the all-important hormone that regulates blood sugar, insulin-resistant cells can stimulate the onset of diabetes and a host of other problems commonly linked to chronic inflammation.

Candida

While inflammation cannot be termed as the root cause of a disease; Candida yeast infection can. Candida Albicans is an opportunistic parasite that resides within your intestinal walls and shares space with other friendly bacteria. Now, while the parasite causes no concern to a healthy gut, a person with a weak gut is likely to be affected by it. You see, an imbalance in the gut almost always leads to an overgrowth of candida. As the parasite multiplies, it tears through the intestinal walls and creates openings for other harmful agents to escape out of the gut, causing infection and inflammation in the process.

Poor diet and Allergens

What you eat, how much eat, and how you eat it can all cause chronic inflammation. A diet that lacks the right amount of nutrients can cause an imbalance in the gut and trigger the onset of a host of intestinal disorders that are closely linked to inflammation. A poor diet can also allow harmful and opportunistic parasites to enter the intestine and cause havoc in it. What's more, if you're allergic to food substances and have been consuming them without your knowledge, you become vulnerable to infections and hence, vulnerable to inflammation too. Consuming a diet that is wholesome, balanced and especially good for you is the first step to avoiding, and even overcoming chronic inflammation.

Diet and Inflammation- Two Sides of the Same Coin

Well lets face it, we live in a world that's heaven to food fanatics who're on a quest for great food- dished out at a fast pace. Blame it on your DNA if it makes you feel better, but an average person can guzzle down a can of coke and demolish a generous serving of crispy potato fries in no time.

From legendary burgers to mouth-watering pizzas, steaks and sandwiches, we are talking about a delicious spread of succulent filling, topped with layers of cheese and fries, stacked one on top of the other – a lip-smacking recipe only a few can refuse!

So, if all is well and everyone is happy then why change- and where does that land us on the health charts?

Well, statistics reveal that what you eat, how much you eat and the way you eat food can all impact your overall health (cliché I know, but true nonetheless). You see, with nearly 20% of our population suffering with problems such as IBS, IBD, heart ailments and Alzheimer's disease, it's become imperative that we address the root cause of them all- chronic inflammation. Now, while I'm not saying that diet is the root cause of all inflammation-related problems, experience has taught me that some diets and foods are generally better tolerated than others.

Continuous v/s Consistent Diet

If you assume, with very little research or knowledge, that sticking to a diet that's fairly constant(and somewhat boring), irrespective of whether you enjoy it or not, will ensure you stay healthy and symptom-free at all times- then you're wrong!

However, sticking to a diet that works for you by embracing foods that aid good health and avoiding foods that aggravate your condition will definitely give you the results you're looking for.

Which is the best diet to follow?

Well, in all honestly, I do not know the answer to this all-important question. Let me also assure you that nobody else knows too. You see, we're all different and seek different things from life. Similarly, we have different digestive systems that respond to foods differently. Let's face it, no one likes to be typecast or forced into a box. So what might work for you might not be necessarily good for me. Conversely, the other way around holds true too.

Therefore, exploring a diet that is known to alleviate symptoms and choosing foods that are especially good for you is the right way of going about things. In essence, you decide- WHAT, WHEN and HOW you want to eat.

The anti-inflammation diet

One of the most common complaints from patients suffering with inflammation is the debilitating discomfort they have to endure on a daily basis. I mean, going to bed after suffering from a painful bout of diarrhea/ constipation or abdominal cramps (the symptoms can be different for different people) while knowing fully well, that you're most likely to endure the same ordeal the next day too can be quite disheartening. While most people perceive prescription and anti-inflammatory drugs as the only solution, some others (the smart ones) explore lifestyle and dietary changes that when combined with medicine give them the results they're looking for. Having explored all of the above combinations, I recommend that you incorporate a balanced mix of the two. You see, while it's important that you continue your current course of medicine, it's equally important that you consume foods that aid better gut-health.

What you need is a complete diet plan that tells what food is good for you and what is not- like the anti-inflammation diet plan. The anti-inflammation diet is a little more than what is generally perceived as a diet. First off, the diet does not particularly target weight loss (although you can lose weight while on it), nor does it recommend you stay on it for a fixed period of time. On the contrary, the anti-inflammation diet has been specifically designed for one purpose- to reduce inflammation and suppress symptoms that are triggered by it.

Based on scientific knowledge, it tells you what foods to consume and what to avoid when you're trying to overcome chronic inflammation. It also shows you ways to select and prepare anti-inflammatory foods- foods that can help reduce inflammation and prevent it from flaring up again. Finally, it works around a holistic approach to give you all-round nutrition and energy. You see, when you are no longer eating foods that are known to cause inflammation, you give yourself a greater chance at fighting the illness and even reversing it sometimes.

Benefits of the anti-inflammation diet

In addition to suppressing symptoms of acute or chronic inflammation, the anti-inflammation diet has been scientifically designed to address and control a host of other secondary conditions that occur as an outcome of inflammation. The diet:

Lowers the risk of heart ailments and reduces bad cholesterol

Given that inflammation is most often the root cause of all other health problems, nipping it in the bud will help strengthen the gut and bounce off any secondary disease. Now, we already know how inflammation weakens the heart and causes heart-related problems. We also know how chronic inflammation can weaken the gut and allow harmful bacteria and bad cholesterol to reside in your body. As these levels of bad cholesterol and bacteria increase, they clog the arteries and prevent it from functioning properly, eventually leading to various heart-related problems. Consuming anti-inflammatory foods not only aid better digestion but also reduce the presence of parasites and bad cholesterol, which in turn lowers the risks of heart ailments.

Helps in weight loss

While the anti-inflammation diet does not target drastic weight loss as its most important deliverable, the fact that you'll be eating only wholesome and healthy foods while on the diet infers that you're most likely to drop those extra kilos over a course of time.

Prevents and controls diabetes

Several years ago, researches identified high levels of inflammation in the bodies of those suffering with type-2 diabetes. You see, as patients with diabetes do not produce enough insulin to regulate the amounts of sugar in their blood, they suffer a greater risk to problems such as obesity and inflammation- both of which are known contributors to type-2 diabetes. Therefore, consuming a diet that prevents the trigger patterns of the disease can ultimately prevent type-2 diabetes too.

Reduces the risk of Cancer, Alzheimer's, and IBS

Prolonged inflammation can injure your body's healthy cells and weaken your immune system. Given that your immune system acts as the backbone for good health, a weak or overactive immune system can cause inflammation in various parts of the body and damage their functionality in the process. As organs become vulnerable to this attack, they become malfunctioned and in the process, lose their ability to deflect serious diseases such as Alzheimer's, Cancer and IBS.

Consuming anti-inflammatory foods will not only reduce inflammation and but also reduce the risk of any injuries to your immune system. With a healthy and functional immune system, you'll have the right tools to deflect IBS and battle even the most serious diseases, including Cancer and Alzheimer's.

The ideal nutritional balance

While we might have different dietary requirements (based on our age, gender and levels of activity), doctors recommend the following dietary strategies and nutritional balances for optimal health. Although it's not imperative that you hold this as a rule-book, it's recommended that you refer to it as a guideline while preparing your meals.

Estimated Caloric Intake

On an average, most adults are required to consume anywhere between 2,000 and 3,000 calories a day. While men and people who are particularly active require additional calories, women and individuals who are less active require fewer calories. Dieticians worldwide recommend that you consume 40-50% of your calories from carbohydrates, 30% from fat, and the remaining 20-30% from proteins. So as a thumb rule, it might help if you consume a small portion of the three foods in each meal. Additionally, a good tip to determine if you're consuming the right amount of calories is to monitor your body weight. If you're consuming the right amount of calories for your activity level, then you should have no problem maintaining your ideal weight.

Your Bowel is *NOT* a Dumping Ground

Most people become anxious or even aggravated when asked to incorporate a change in their eating habits; worse if they're asked to avoid or eliminate their favourite foods. In fact, I often hear hallmark responses such as "But surely, I must be allowed to eat bread- It's my staple food and I could never feel full-enough without it" and "But sugar makes me feel good and gives me energy- I believe I need it".

Well, if truth be told- you don't!

You see, if you've been experiencing symptoms of chronic inflammation, then there's a good chance that they'll manifest into some more alarming if you don't take the necessary steps to treat it. Consuming foods that have repeatedly given you symptoms will only aggravate your levels of inflammation. On the contrary, eliminating foods that are harmful to your condition and incorporating foods that are anti-inflammatory can help you nip inflammation in its bud.

Allergy or Intolerance- Know your sore points

The terms food intolerance and allergy can mean different things to different people. In essence, allergens are foods that act as your trigger factors- foods that stimulate an immediate inflammatory response, irrespective of the portions you have them in. An allergic response to food usually occurs when your body's immune system recognizes it as potentially harmful.

On the contrary, food intolerance is not triggered by an alert or an overactive immune system. In fact, most often, large quantities of intolerant-food has to be ingested for it to trigger a response. Sometimes however, you can become sensitive to foods that cause food intolerance. For instance, some people can be sensitive to particular foods because they lack the right digestive enzymes to digest it- so if you lack the digestive enzyme lactase; you're most likely to be lactose intolerant. Some other common intolerants are vasoactive amines and monosodium glutamate, also known as MSG.

Testing for allergies and food intolerance

While there are a wide range of tests that "claim" to identify and differentiate allergens from food-intolerance, very few of them have shown substantial proof to validate their claim. Your best bet is to stay tuned to your body's responses. Remember that you-are-your-best-judge. So if you feel that you're particularly allergic or intolerant to certain foods, have it in restricted quantities first to rule out any assumptions. However, if the responses persist, stop consuming it.

Some foods that are known to cause inflammation are:

Sugar

Foods that are high in sugar tend to be high in calories and low in essential nutrients. While they might be delicious ingredients to include into your favourite recipes, processed sugars contain cytokines that trigger the release of inflammatory responses in your body.

Saturated Fats

Foods that are rich in saturated fats trigger fat tissues called adipose that are known to cause inflammation. In addition to inflammation, foods rich in saturated fat (such as pizzas, cheese, red meat, full-fat dairy products, pasta and grain-based desserts) are also known to trigger the onset of a host of diseases such as heart ailments, arthritis inflammation, obesity and even cancer.

Trans-fat

Most processed foods contain trans-fat or artificial fat and are injected with hydrogen oils for a firmer appearance. These fats can be found in most processed and fried foods and are known to be the most potent triggers for intestinal inflammation. Some foods that are rich in trans-fat are frozen foods, processed foods, cookies, donuts, and crackers.

Caffeine

As a stimulant, caffeine can give you the "kick" you need to get through a long and busy day. However, it also acts as an irritant to the bowel and can trigger inflammation. What's more, excessive amounts of caffeine can exacerbate symptoms of IBS and IBD patients.

Alcohol

Alcohol is another irritant that is known to trouble the bowel and cause inflammation. It can also contribute to diarrhea, abdominal discomfort and indigestion (also recognized as heartburn).

Refined Carbohydrates

Considering you're on a 2,000-calorie-a-day diet, adult women are advised to consume anywhere between 160 to 200 grams of carbohydrates a day. On the contrary, adult men can consume anywhere between 240 to 300 grams of carbohydrates a day. However, a majority of this should be consumed in the form of healthy carbohydrates- foods that are particularly less-refined, less-processed and low on glycemic. Foods made out of white flour, white rice and white potatoes are considered to be sources of refined carbohydrates. These high-glycemic foods increase the production of glycation which in turn causes inflammation in the gut.

Mono-sodium glutamate

As discussed before, Mono-sodium glutamate (MSG) is a flavor-enhancing food additive that's most commonly used in Asian cuisine. The substance is a known ingredient in most oriental foods and can trigger chronic inflammation if consumed often enough.

Gluten and Casein

Common allergens like gluten and casein (proteins found in dairy and wheat) are known to promote symptoms of inflammation. In essence, Gluten is the name given to the protein found in wheat, rye and barley. Casein, on the other hand, is found in most whey protein products. People suffering with celiac disease (mainly caused by an allergy to Gluten) should follow a diet that is strictly gluten-free.

In pursuit of a symptom-free life

Cutting back on foods that are known to alleviate inflammatory responses and paying attention to your meal patterns can help you go from symptom-prone to symptom-free. While I stress on the need to follow a consistent diet, I ask you not to skip meals at any cost. Following a balanced diet that includes appropriate portions of the recommended foods holds the key to winning the battle against inflammation.

Dietary Therapies

Case study- The experience of a dear friend

Ethan's digestion had been upset for three years, ever since he suffered an attack of acute diarrhea, barely a day before his 24th birthday. In addition to diarrhea, he complained of bloating, abdominal cramps, and discomfort after eating certain foods. While initial diagnosis revealed no particular problem, a comprehensive gastroenterological diagnosis, done after the problem persisted for several more weeks, revealed that he had severe inflammation around his intestinal lining and a type of intestinal bowel disease called Crohn's disease.

As the condition had been left undetected and untreated for long, it soon manifested into symptoms such as painful defecation along with mucus and pus in stools. Upon detection, Ethan was hastily put on anti-inflammatory drugs to reduce inflammation and immunosuppressants to prevent his overactive immune system from triggering further inflammation. While the drugs did provide some relief, Ethan continued to experience discomfort after eating certain foods- something that would immediately put him into relapse. It was only then that he was diagnosed to be particularly intolerant to certain foods. In fact, doctors revealed that it was his body's allergic reaction to intolerant foods that triggered the painful bouts.

Doctors advised him to observe his body's responses to the foods he consumed. This was his learning curve- he'd consume a variety of food choices and would make a note of foods that made him feel uncomfortable. Not wanting to discard an otherwise important food source, he spent time over his meals and would chew on his food slowly. He also repeated the process until he was certain he was allergic to certain foods. Over a period of time, he became aware of the anti-inflammation diet and through it, learnt of ways to suppress his symptoms even before they threatened to appear. Today, he leads an active life and has learnt to prolong his periods of remission with diet and medicine.

Beating Inflammation with the right kind of food

When the lining of your intestine is inflamed or swollen, you're likely to experience a lot of discomfort- abdominal pain, irritation in the stomach, irregular bowel movements, irritation while defecating as well as occasional mucus or blood in stools are some of the symptoms patients usually complain of while being diagnosed with inflammation. While these symptoms might vary in frequency depending on the severity of the inflammation, if left ignored, they can become progressively painful and uncomfortable. If you're hoping to reverse the signs of inflammation, then it's important that you consume foods that help restore gut-flora and fight inflammation.

You see, in addition to giving up allergic foods that trigger irritation, it's important that you also include foods that ease discomfort and help suppress inflammation. Below are some foods that help fight inflammation- foods that I've tried and continue to swear by. I urge you to try them too.

Animal-based Omega-3 fatty acids

Now, unlike Omega-6 fatty acids, which are consumed in relatively large quantities, omega-3 fatty acids are often secluded from our diets. The type of fat has exceptional anti-inflammatory properties and does wonders to heal an ailing and imbalanced gut. In fact, nutritionists recommend that patients with chronic inflammation should double their regular consumption of the fat so as to aid speedy recovery. Oily fish including sardines and salmon as well as speciality eggs are some of the foods rich in animal-based omega-3 fatty acids.

Dark Leafy Greens

As discussed before, cytokine is a type of protein that triggers inflammation in the gut. Given that vitamin E is known to prevent the immune system from secreting this protein; it makes sense that we consume foods that are rich in the particular vitamin. Leafy greens, especially the ones that are particularly dark, such as spinach, and broccoli are excellent sources of vitamin E. The carotenoids and flavonoids responsible for their color are antioxidants by nature and are excellent at fighting inflammation.

Berries

Berries contain high levels of ellagic acid, also known to fight inflammation. They're anti-oxidant by nature and help cut the risk of cardio-vascular diseases by reducing the amount of bad LDL cholesterol in the bloodstream. As high levels of bad LDL is known to trigger conditions that are linked to inflammation, consuming a variety of berries including blueberries, strawberries, acai Berries, goji Berries and blackberries can help control inflammation and promote general health.

Tea

Now, we all know that green tea is packed with antioxidants that help reverse the signs of inflammation, ageing and an ailing gut. What many people don't know is that in addition to green tea, other herbal tea infusions such as chamomile and hibiscus too contain anti-inflammatory properties that are great for your gut.

Gut Healing Probiotic Foods

As discussed before, your gut is home to a large number of living organisms, nearly 100 trillion of them that form the all-important intestinal flora. Now ideally, the ratio between good and opportunistic bacteria should be 85:15, with the good bacteria overpowering the opportunistic ones by a long shot. However, people with weak guts and intestinal diseases suffer an imbalance in this ratio. In such cases, the opportunistic bacteria outnumber the good ones, causing inflammation and a host of other problems that are linked to it.

As probiotics foods are essentially made up of good bacteria and yeast, consuming foods that are rich in probiotics can help promote the growth of good bacteria in your gut, in the process reversing and even maintaining the ideal ratio soon enough. Fermented foods and probiotic supplements that are readily available in market today are great sources of probiotics.

Home-cooked bone broth

Looking at a bone, it's hard to think of it as nutritious. In fact, most people are tempted to discard it right away. However, if you're suffering from inflammation or a weak gut, then it's advised that you hold onto those hard-shells and make broth out of them. In addition to being anti-inflammatory, bone broth is packed with proteins, minerals and vitamins that aid in healing a weak and inflamed gut. They're also known to strengthen bones and act as excellent detoxification agents. What's more, they also contain amino acids such as glycine and glutamine, both of which are excellent for weak guts.

Fermentable fibres such as sweet potatoes

Sweet potatoes belong to the family of the morning glory plant and are different from yams, with which they are commonly confused. They are packed with nutrients and are rich in dietary fibre, beta-carotene, vitamin C, manganese, vitamin N6, potassium and iron- all of which work wonders to reduce inflammation. While there are different varieties of sweet potatoes- all of which are beneficial, the purple colored sweet potato is believed to provide the highest levels of anti-oxidant and anti-inflammatory activity.

Fermented Foods

Fermented foods are foods that have been put through a process called lacto fermentation, in which natural bacteria is allowed to feed on the sugar and starch present in food so as to create lactic acid. Now, in addition to acting as a preservative, the process gives birth to beneficial enzymes, B-vitamins, Omega-3 fatty acids and other probiotics that help heal and soothe an inflamed gut. Foods such as Sauerkraut and kimchi are some examples of fermented foods.

Shitake mushrooms

Shiitake mushrooms have proved to be excellent for reducing inflammation, bad bacteria, harmful viruses, and ironically even fungus. The type of fungus is also rich in B vitamins and antioxidants that aid in supporting a weak and ailing gut.

Garlic

Garlic is an anti-fungal agent and is known to be highly effective in the treatment of inflammation and candida yeast infection. It's also known to reduce bad cholesterol, heal ulcers and improve digestion.

Some other food sources

Finally, in addition to the above sources, it's recommended that you consume a good mix of the following foods so as to reduce any inflammation and stay symptom-free.

- Foods such as Nuts, seeds and legumes (chai seeds, cashew nuts, almonds, walnuts, chickpeas & lentils)
- Fresh vegetables and fruits
- Anti-inflammatory herbs and spices such as cinnamon, cloves, thyme, oregano, pumpkin pie spice mixture, marjoram, and sage
- Plenty of water and healthy fluids

Note:

Here's a quick thumb rule that's applicable to all diets. The foods that I've mentioned so far will tell you what to avoid, what to reduce and what to eliminate from your diet. If you're in doubt and want to know if the food you wish to consume is in the allowed or avoid list, then I urge you to look at the ingredients to recognize the family of food they fall under. While the foods don't promise to cure the condition in anyway, its main intention is to have the symptoms under control, thereby facilitating for a more comfortable lifestyle.

Beyond anti-inflammation and Paleo diets

The Mediterranean diet plan

On a side note, if you're particularly comfortable with diets such as the anti-inflammation and the Paleo diet plan and are keen to explore other healthy options, then the Mediterranean diet might be right for you. The diet, similar to the other two diets works at eliminating known trigger-foods and incorporating foods that aid in building a healthy gut. A style that has its roots in the countries bordering the Mediterranean sea, this diet emphasises on:

- Consuming predominately foods such as fresh fruits and vegetables, whole grains, pulses and nuts

- Substituting butter with healthy fats such as olive oil

- Substituting salt with herbs and spices

- Restricting the consumption of red meat to the bare minimum

- Consuming fish and poultry at least twice a week

The Gluten- free diet plan

A gluten-free diet is a plan that strictly eliminates the protein gluten from your diet. As Gluten is predominantly found in grains such as wheat, barley, and rye, the diet does not allow the consumption of them. While the diet is perhaps the most difficult to follow, it's known to be especially good for people suffering from Celiac disease (a condition that is allergic to gluten-based foods). Given that the diet is known to instantly reduce the symptoms present in patients with Celiac disease, incorporating the diet and following it strictly is an effort worth making.

Eating to Beat Inflammation

Building a healthy pantry

Some people cling on to the idea that a nutritious meal must include a combination of protein and starch, such as steak pie- cabbage- potatoes -and -gravy or fish-peas- and chips (old fashion I know, but not necessarily right for you). Now, although these foods are widely accepted, recent research has revealed that starch found in foods such as bread- potato- sugar, and protein found in foods such as eggs- meat- fish-and -poultry require different gastric juices for complete digestion. So, when foods such as these are eaten together, there's a conflict between the gastric juices and neither food is likely to be digested fully. What's worse is that the conflict triggers a chemical reaction that results in symptoms such as indigestion, bloating, gas and even inflammation. You see, not only is it unnecessary to eat this way, but it also puts a lot of stress on your digestive system- something I'm sure you'd prefer to avoid. The Anti-inflammatory meal plan that I've listed below takes away the guess work, leaving you with healthy and delicious recipes for two whole weeks.

Dietary tips for healthy living

Consistency is the Key

While you might be tempted to eliminate various food types all at once, I urge not to do exactly so. The idea is to ease your system into the plan; not shock and drive it away to a point of no return. Take things slow and easy at first. Avoid few foods that are bad for you while simultaneously incorporating food choices that are good- one at a time. Remember that following the diet should feel like a way of life. Given that it's going to be a life-long process; you'll have all the time to ease yourself into it. What's important is that you maintain consistency at all times.

Follow regular meal patterns

It's important to have regular meals throughout the day. Missing meals and then snacking on high-fat foods can lead to bloating, gas, indigestion and inflammation in the long run.

Chew on your meals- Remember to taste your food

Eating quickly or rushing through meals can lead to belching or indigestion. Make sure you take time over your meals and enjoy it too.

Getting Started- Building a 14- day plan

Now, for all those who're in a hurry, I've created a special meal plan that takes away the guess work from you. Alternatively, you can also mix and match to create a meal plan that suits your palate the best.

Note:

The recipes for the below meal plan are listed in the following chapters.

Week 1

Day	Breakfast	Lunch	Dinner
1	Mixed grain porridge	Apple-laced pasta with chicken sausage	Allspice rice mix
2	Orzo with almonds and blueberries	Chicken burger with applesauce	Chicken with steamed broccoli
3	Cinnamon and apple crepes	Vegetable and chicken salad	Chicken Casserole
4	Fruit and protein smoothie	Orzo with chicken and tomato sauce	Beetroot and blue cheese risotto
5	Oatmeal with pumpkin spice mix	Pasta salad	Bulgar rice with mixed roots
6	Blueberry and cottage cheese pie	Barbequed chicken salad	Garbanzo bean with turkey salad
7	Berries with ricotta oatmeal	Chicken and black bean salad	Pear soup with toasted bread

Week 2

Day	Breakfast	Lunch	Dinner
1	American cinnamon pancakes	Broiled chicken with blue cheese	Root veg salad
2	Minty avocado smoothie	Chicken chow Mein with spaghetti sauce	Baked fish
3	Carrot and chickpea soup	Chicken soup with fruit salad	Baked chicken with vegetables
4	Blueberries with greek yogurt	Coconut rice	Mixed rice
5	Orzo with fruit and yogurt	Spinach with tofu	Grilled chicken with vegetables
6	Quick cheese bread	Vegetable salad with blue cheese	Tofu soup
7	Honeyed granola	Egg salad with choice of bread	Grilled chicken salad

Breakfast Recipes

1. Mixed grain porridge

Ingredients

- 50 g bucket wheat flakes
- 50 g quinoa flakes
- 50 g millet flakes
- 600 ml semi-skimmed milk
- 300 ml water
- 2 bananas
- 4 tablespoons greek yogurt
- A drizzle organic honey
- A sprinkle cinnamon power, to serve

Instructions

1. Put the grain flakes, milk and water into a saucepan and bring it to a boil
2. Mash one banana and slice the other. Blend the mashed banana into the porridge
3. Spoon into a bowl
4. Top it with yogurt, sliced banana, a drizzle of honey and a sprinkle of cinnamon powder

2. Orzo with almonds and blueberries

Ingredients

- 1 1/2 cups Water
- 3/4 cup organic orzo
- 1/2 cup whole blueberries

- 2/3 cup semi-skimmed Milk
- 1 tbsp almond butter
- 1 1/4 tsps flavoured extract
- 1/2 tsp cinnamon powder
- 2 tbsps low at yogurt
- A drizzle organic honey

Instructions

1. Boil orzo in a medium-sized pan, stirring until water is fully absorbed
2. Turn off heat.
3. Drop in blueberries, milk, almond butter, flavoured extract and cinnamon powder
4. Split into 2 bowls, topping it with a dollop of yogurt

3. Cinnamon and apple crepes

Ingredients

- 1/2 cup beaten egg white
- 1/3 cup organic soy flour
- 1 tbsp olive oil
- 1 cup semi-skimmed milk
- 1 peeled and chopped apple
- 1/3 cup unsweetened applesauce
- 2/3 cup cooked oatmeal
- 1/4 tsp cinnamon powder
- 2 slices bacon

Instructions

1. In a small mixing bowl, blend egg whites, flour, oil and milk to form a batter of medium-thick consistency

2. Grease two crepe pans with cooking oil

3. Add a quarter of the batter in the pan. Pour enough batter to make one crepe

4. Close the pan with a lid and wait for it to turn golden brown in color

5. Flip it over and cook the second side for a minute

6. Sauté cooked oatmeal, bacon and cinnamon until tender to make filling

7. Place the filling inside the crepe and fold three sides

8. Add a drizzle of apple sauce and serve

4. Fruit and protein smoothie

Ingredients

- 3 Egg whites that have been hard- boiled the night before
- 1 Apple
- 1 cup Strawberries
- 1 1/2 tbsps of raw ginger (optional)
- 2 tbsps raw almonds
- 1 tsp olive oil

Instructions

1. Blend all ingredients together until they are of a chunky cereal consistency and serve

5. Oatmeal with pumpkin spice mix

Ingredients

- 3 cups water

- 3/4 cup oats
- 2 tsps pumpkin Spice
- 2 scoops protein powder of your choice
- 1 cup organic honey
- Some halved walnuts

Instructions

1. Boil pumpkin spice mix and oats in a medium-sized pan.
2. Blend in the protein powder.
3. Stir in honey and serve with walnuts

6. Blueberry and cottage cheese pie

Ingredients

- 3/4 cup low fat cottage cheese
- 1 tsp olive oil
- 1/2 cup organic applesauce
- 1/2 cup blueberries
- 5 tsp crushed almonds

Instructions

1. Place cottage cheese, olive oil, and applesauce in a bowl.
2. Mix them all together
3. Serve with blueberries and almonds

7. Berries with ricotta oatmeal

Ingredients

- 14g any protein powder of your choice
- 3/4 cup cooked oatmeal

- 1/2 cup assorted berries
- 1/4 cup low-fat ricotta cheese
- 2 tbsps of crushed almonds
- 1/2 cup semi-skimmed milk

Instructions

1. Blend in protein powder with milk and add it into previously cooked oatmeal

2. Drop in your choice of berries and cook for 2 minutes

3. Stir in some low-fat ricotta cheese and serve with crushed almonds

8. American cinnamon pancakes

Ingredients

- 250 g fresh or frozen fruits
- 2 tbsps water
- 40 g cornmeal
- 40 g tapioca flour
- ½ tsp ground cinnamon
- 200 ml low fat yogurt
- 1 egg
- 1 tbsp sunflower oil
- Greek yogurt, to serve
- Organic honey, to serve

Instructions

1. Simmer the fruits with water in a medium-sized pan

2. Sift in flours and cinnamon in a separate bowl

3. Whisk egg and yogurt into the mixture to make smooth batter

4. Light heat a non-stick griddle

5. Drop in spoonful's of batter and cook them until golden brown on both sides

6. Place the pancake on a plate

7. Serve it with fruit mixture, yogurt and honey

9. Minty avocado smoothie

Ingredients

- 1 ripe avocado
- 3 stems of mint
- Juice of 1 lime
- 450 ml apple juice

Instructions

1. Blend the flesh of one avocado with mint, lime juice and half the apple juice.

2. Add the remaining apple juice

3. Pour into glass and serve cold

10. Carrot and chickpea soup

Ingredients

- 1 tbsp sunflower oil
- 1 large onion, chopped
- 500 g of diced carrots
- 1 tsp cinnamon powder
- 1 tsp fennel seeds
- 1 clove garlic, chopped

- 1 tsp chopped ginger

- 410 g canned chickpeas, drained

- litres gluten and wheat free vegetable stock

- 300 ml semi-skimmed milk

- Salk and pepper to taste

- Chopped parsley

Instructions

1. Sauté onions, carrots, ground spices, garlic and ginger until cooked

2. Mix in chickpeas, stock and simmer for 30 minutes

3. Puree the soup in batches until smooth

4. Add milk and reheat gently

5. Garnish with fresh parsley and serve with warm bread

11. Blueberries with Greek yogurt

Ingredients

- 1 cup Strawberries

- 3/4 cup Blueberries

- 1 cup low-fat Greek yogurt

- 2 tbsps chopped walnuts

Instructions

1. Stir fruit and nuts into yogurt

2. Serve cold

12. Orzo with fruit and yogurt

Ingredients

- 1/3 cup Orzo

- 1/2 cup semi-skimmed milk
- 1/2 cup water
- 1/2 tbsp organic honey
- 1 tsp vanilla extract
- 1/4 tsp pumpkin pie spice mix
- 3 tbsps low-fat Greek yogurt
- 1/4 cup chopped strawberries
- 1 tbsp crushed almonds

Instructions

1. Simmer orzo, milk, water, preserves, vanilla and pumpkin spice mix under medium flame
2. Cook uncovered until thick
3. Sprinkle extra pumpkin spice mix and serve with crushed almonds

13. Quick cheese bread

Ingredients

- 250 g gluten and wheat free bread flour with natural gum
- ½ tsp salt
- 1 tsp gluten-free mustard powder
- 100 g mature cheddar cheese
- 300 ml semi-skimmed milk
- 2 eggs
- 50 g reduced fat spread
- 1 tbsp sesame seeds

Instructions

1. Put all the dry ingredients into a mixing bowl. Add cheese.

2. Mix in milk, eggs, melted spread along with the dry ingredients and stir until smooth

3. Pour the mixture into a lightly oiled loaf tin

4. Bake in a preheated oven at 180D C for 30 minutes

5. Leave to cool

6. Serve warm, cold or toasted

14. Honeyed granola

Ingredients

- 3 tbsp clear honey

- 3 tbsp sunflower oil

- 50 g porridge oats

- 50 g miller or quinoa flakes

- 50 g mixed seeds

- 50 g assorted nuts

Instructions

1. Warm the honey and oil in a pan

2. Mix in the remaining ingredients

3. Tip the mixture into lightly oiled tin

4. Bake in a preheated over at 180D C for 6 minutes

5. Leave to cool and serve

Lunch recipes

1. Apple-laced pasta with chicken sausage

Ingredients

- 2/3 cup cooked pasta
- 1/2 tsp olive oil
- 2 tbsp cooking wine
- 1 chopped onion
- 1/2 link of slicked chicken sausage
- 1/4 cup chopped apple
- 1 cup baby spinach leaves

Instructions

1. Heat oil and wine in a non-stick pan
2. Sauté sausage and cook for 2 minutes
3. Stir in diced apples, spinach and pasta.
4. Add additional water if required and cook for 2 minutes.
5. Serve warm

2. Chicken burger with applesauce

Ingredients

- 1/3 cup home-cooked applesauce
- 3 tbsps cooked granulated oats
- 1/2 tsp red chilli powder
- 3 oz minced chicken breast
- Spinach Salad

- 1 1/2 tsps olive oil
- 2 tsps lemon juice
- 2 tsps Water
- 2 slices chopped onion
- 2 egg white
- 1/2 Tomato, chopped
- 1/2 cup Strawberries

Instructions

1. Mix 1/4 cup applesauce, oatmeal, egg whites and onions. Add minced chicken and shape into burger

2. Heat non-stick griddle and grill the burger patties until cooked

3. Place the cooked chicken on a plate. Drizzle applesauce.

4. In a separate bowl, mix applesauce and oatmeal to get right consistency.

5. Additionally, mix spinach, tomato and strawberries in a salad bowl and squeeze in a dash of lime

6. Serve all three together for a complete meal

3. Vegetable and chicken salad

Ingredients

- 1 1/2 tsps olive oil
- 3 tbsps lemon juice
- 1 tsp pepper
- 2 cups ripped lettuce
- 1 cup Strawberries, sliced

- 1 1/2 cups diced cucumber
- 1 cup halved cherry tomatoes
- 1/2 cup diced mushrooms
- 250 g diced and cooked chicken breast
- Crushed croutons

Instructions

1. Whisk the first three ingredients in a bowl to make a dressing
2. Make a salad with the remaining ingredients
3. Serve with croutons and dressing

4. Orzo with chicken and tomato sauce

Ingredients

- 1/3 cup orzo
- 1 1/2 tsp olive oil
- 1/8 medium-sized onion, chopped
- 1/2 clove minced garlic
- 1/4 cup tomato puree
- 1/4 cup water
- 4 oz vegetable broth
- 1/2 tsp bay leaves
- 1/2 tsp dried oregano
- 1/2 cup chopped green beans
- 1/4 cup chicken breast, chopped
- Salt & Pepper

Instructions

1. Cook orzo and set aside

2. Sauté onions and garlic in1/2 tsp of oil over medium to high heat

3. Mix in tomato puree, water, broth, bay leaves, and oregano and stir well

4. Season with Salt & Pepper and bring to a boil

5. Drop in beans and cook for another 8 minutes

6. Sauté chicken until cooked

7. Add orzo and drizzle olive oil

8. Serve warm

5. Pasta salad

Ingredients

- Cooked pasta
- 7 cherry tomatoes
- 1/2 oz low-fat cheese (cubed)
- 1/2 green bell pepper
- 1 tsp olive oil
- 1 tbsp lemon juice
- 1 tsp garlic power
- 3 tbsp black olives
- 1 tsp Italian seasoning
- Salt and pepper

Instructions

1. Whisk olive oil, lemon juice, garlic powder, Italian seasoning, salt and pepper together in a bowl

2. Stir in cooked pasta with tomatoes, cheese, and black olives

3. Coat pasta with salad dressing and serve

6. Barbequed chicken salad

Ingredients

- 2 tsps olive oil
- 3 oz diced chicken breast
- 1 1/2 cups diced peppers
- 1/4 cup diced onions
- 1/8 tsp apple cider vinegar
- 1/8 tsp barbeque sauce
- 1 tsp minced garlic
- 2 cups coleslaw mix
- Salt and pepper

Instructions

1. Sauté chicken breast, pepper, onion, vinegar, barbeque sauce and garlic until chicken is cooked

2. Serve the chicken mix with coleslaw mix

3. Black bean with avocado and turkey

7. Chicken and black bean salad

Ingredients

- 1/2 cup canned and drained black beans
- 1 diced red bell pepper
- 2 cups zucchini
- 1 1/2 cups diced red onions

- 1/2 cup diced avocado
- 1/2 tsp cumin powder
- 1 tbsp balsamic vinegar
- 1 tbsp lime juice
- 2 tbsps chopped parsley
- 1 tbsp dry oregano
- Salt and pepper - to taste
- 1 tsp Tabasco Sauce - or to taste
- 4 oz leftover(cooked) turkey breast
- 1/3 cup Low-fat cheese

Instructions

1. Combine all ingredients except cheese

2. Mix in Tabasco sauce and salt and pepper to taste

3. Serve with grated cheese

8. Broiled chicken with blue cheese

Ingredients

- 10 cups Baby spinach
- 2 cups thinly-sliced celery
- 2 oz Low-fat blue cheese
- 3 tbsps sun-dried tomatoes
- 2 tbsps lemon juice
- 6 oz broiled-cooked and shredded chicken breast
- 1 tbsp cooking oil
- 1/4 tbsp Ground black pepper

- 1 tbsp Dijon mustard

Instructions

1. Mix salad ingredients with lemon juice and set aside

2. Season already cooked broiled chicken with pepper, Dijon mustard and sauté for 1 minute in oil-greased pan

3. Once warm, mix the salad ingredients and chicken mixture in a serving bowl

4. Sprinkle blue cheese and serve

9. Chicken chow Mein with spaghetti sauce

Ingredients

- 14 oz minced chicken breast
- 2 1/2 tbsps olive oil
- 1 cup sliced mushrooms
- 4 oz minced lemon grass
- 1 tbsp chopped jalapeno pepper
- 1 cup minced scallions
- 2 tbsps minced fresh parsley
- 3 tbsps hoisin sauce
- 3 cups cooked spaghetti squash

Instructions

1. Sauté minced chicken in 1 tablespoon of olive oil until well cooked

2. Add mushrooms, lemon grass, jalapeno, scallions, parsley and stir in hoisin sauce

3. Place the mixture on a bed of cooked spaghetti squash and serve

10. Chicken soup with fruit salad

Ingredients

- 2 cups basic unsalted chicken stock
- 1 cup leftover cooked chicken breast
- 2 carrots, chopped
- 2 stocks celery, chopped
- 4 oz diced zucchini
- 1 clove minced garlic
- salt and pepper, to taste
- 3 tsps olive oil
- 2 cups strawberries
- 1 cup blueberries
- 1/2 cup fat-free whipped cream

Instructions

1. Boil the stock in a large pot

2. Add the next 6 ingredients and simmer all together under low flame for 20 minutes

3. Season with salt and pepper

4. Drizzle 1 1/2 teaspoon olive oil and set aside

To make the fruit salad:

1. Mix berries with whipped cream and serve

11. Coconut Rice

Ingredients

- 1 cup cooked rice
- 2 tbsp cooking oil
- 1 tsp minced garlic
- 1/4 cup chopped red bell pepper
- 1 tbsp minced jalapeno pepper
- 1/4 tsp dried thyme
- Salt to taste
- 2 tbsps coconut milk
- 1/4 cup canned and rinsed kidney beans
- 2 minced scallions

Instructions

1. Sauté garlic and pepper under flame
2. Add the jalapeno, fresh thyme, and salt, stirring often, about 1 minute, until fragrant
3. Add coconut milk and bring the mixture to a boil
4. Sauté beans until cooked
5. Add cooked rice and remove from heat
6. Sprinkle minced scallions and serve

12. Spinach with tofu

Ingredients

- 10 cups baby spinach cut into bite-sized pieces
- 1 tbsp olive oil
- 1/2 tsp Cumin
- 2 tbsps Soy sauce

- 2 tbsps Minced hot chillies
- 1 tbsp Minced ginger
- 10 oz tofu
- Salt and pepper - to taste
- 3 oz Low-fat cream cheese
- 1/4 cup chopped parsley

Instructions

1. Sauté cumin, soy sauce, chillies, ginger, and tofu with salt and pepper

2. Add the cream cheese, parsley, curry powder, and spinach

3. Serve warm

13. Vegetable salad with blue cheese

Ingredients

- Mix pack of salad vegetables (cucumber, iceberg lettuce, carrots)
- Blue cheese
- Choice of dressing sauce
- Toasted croutons
- Toasted bread of your choice (non-wheat and gluten based)

Instructions

1. Mix salad ingredients with dressing sauce

2. Sprinkle blue cheese and croutons

3. Serve with toasted bread

14. Egg salad with choice of bread

Ingredients:

- 1 tsp extra virgin olive oil
- 1 cup chopped onions
- 3/4 cup cooked peas
- 4 eggs, beaten
- 1 tsp Parmesan cheese, grated
- salt and pepper - to taste

Instructions

1. Stir fry onions and peas until cooked

2. Reduce heat; add eggs, salt and pepper

3. Scramble and sauté eggs until cooked

4. Remove from flame and add cheese

5. Serve hot and with your choice of bread

Dinner Recipes

1. Allspice rice mix

Ingredients

- 1/3 cup cooked rice
- 1 tsp cooking oil
- 1 cup diced onion
- 1 tbsp coconut milk
- 1/4 tsp allspice mix
- Shopped cilantro
- Salt & pepper to taste

Instructions

1. Sauté onions until translucent
2. Add allspice mix and 1 tbsp coconut milk
3. Stir under low flame and set aside
4. Add sautéed onion mixture to cooked rice
5. Sprinkle with cilantro and serve

2. Chicken with steamed broccoli

Ingredients

- 3 oz sliced chicken breast
- 2 cups steamed broccoli
- 1/2 tsps olive oil
- 1 cup chopped green bell pepper
- 1 cup chopped red bell pepper
- 3/4 cup chopped onion

- 1 clove minced garlic
- 1 cup halved cherry tomatoes
- Salt and pepper to taste
- 2 tsp Sliced almonds

Instructions

1. Steam broccoli and set aside
2. Sauté chicken, green pepper, red pepper, onion, and garlic until they're cooked
3. Toss in tomatoes and steamed broccoli
4. Garnish with almonds and serve

3. Chicken Casserole

Ingredients

- 4.5 cups cooked pasta
- 1 tbsp olive oil
- 5 oz ground turkey breast
- 4 cups canned tomatoes
- 1 cup chopped onion
- 16 oz chopped vegetables
- 26 oz tomato sauce
- 1 cup water
- 1 tsp Italian seasoning
- to taste salt and pepper
- 3/4 cup mozzarella cheese

Instructions

1. Sauté turkey, tomatoes, bell pepper and onion until cooked

2. Add vegetables, tomato sauce, water, spices, salt and pepper and cook for 15 minutes

3. Mix in cooked pasta and cheese

4. Pour mixture in greased baking tin and bake for 25 minutes at 180D C

5. Drizzle olive oil and serve

4. Beetroot and blue cheese risotto

Ingredients

- 1 tbsp olive oil
- 1 cup chopped onion
- 2 cup chopped beetroot
- 200 g risotto
- Italian seasoning
- Salt and pepper
- Few sage leaves
- 2 litres of gluten-free vegetable stock
- 125 g of grated blue cheese

Instructions

1. Sauté onions and beetroot until cooked

2. Stir in the pasta and cook for 5 minutes

3. Add sage, seasoning, and stock and cook for 15 minutes

4. Stir in cheese, stir till melted and serve

5. Bulgar rice with mixed roots

Ingredients

- 1 tbsp olive oil
- 1 cup chopped red onion
- 150 g of diced parsnip
- 200 g of diced carrots
- 4 cloves
- 1 tsp cinnamon powder
- 1 tsp paprika
- 410 g green lentils
- 125 g bulgar rice
- 1 tbsp tomato puree
- Salt and pepper
- 900 of gluten-free vegetable stock

Instructions

1. Sauté onions, spices lentils, bulgar rice, tomato puree, seasoning, vegetable stock and bring to a boil
2. Let the mixture of 25 minutes under low flame until cooked
3. Spoon into bowls and serve

6. Garbanzo bean with turkey salad

Ingredients

- 1 1/2 heads of shredded iceberg lettuce
- 2 cups sliced celery
- 3/4 cup sliced carrots
- 3 cups diced mushrooms
- 1 cup diced onions

- 3/4 cup canned and drained garbanzo beans
- 2 oz light tuna
- 2 oz skimmed-mozzarella cheese
- 3 oz diced turkey
- 2 tsp crushed dried basil
- 3 tsp olive oil
- 1/4 cup low-Fat dressing of your choice

Instructions

1. Arrange celery, carrots, mushrooms, onions, red pepper and garbanzo beans on a plate of lettuce
2. Sauté chicken until cooked, adding seasoning to taste
3. Add tuna and cheese and cook until cheese melts.
4. Crush basil
5. Drizzle dressing, olive oil and serve

7. Pear soup

Ingredients

- 2 tbsp butter
- 2 peeled and coarsely chopped pears
- 1 cup chopped onion
- 6 cups gluten-free chicken stock or bone broth
- 1/2 cup coconut cream
- fresh thyme
- Salt & pepper
- Black seed oil

Instructions

1. Sauté onions in butter until translucent

2. Add pear and sauté for 5 minutes

3. Drop in chicken stock, salt, pepper, thyme, coconut cream, black seed oil and simmer for 10 times under low flame

4. Remove from flame, blend into puree and strain

5. Simmer the strained mixture until it's of the right consistency

6. Serve with toasted bread

8. Root veg salad

Ingredients

- 2 cups chopped carrots

- 2 cups chopped beetroots

- 1 cup Pomegranate

- ½ cup of mixed pumpkin and sunflower seeds

For Dressing:

- 2 tbsp apple cider vinegar

- 3 tbsp olive oil

- 2 tbsp lemon juice

- Crushed cilantro leaves

- Salt and pepper to taste

Instructions

1. Add all the salad ingredients in a large bowl

2. Toss in the dressing ingredients

3. Season with salt and pepper

4. Serve with warm bread

9. Baked fish

Ingredients

- 2 tbsp olive oil
- 3 oz oily fish (salmon or sardines)
- 1 1/2 cups sliced summer squash
- 1 1/2 cups sliced zucchini
- 3/4 cup sliced bell pepper
- 3/4 cup sliced tomato
- Salt and pepper - to taste

Instructions

1. Preheat oven at 350°F
2. Place fish and vegetables in a baking tray
3. Sprinkle salt and pepper
4. Add salt and pepper
5. Drizzle with olive oil and bake for 10 minutes
6. Serve with choice of bread

10. Baked chicken with vegetables

Ingredients

- 4 cups pre-cooked cauliflower
- 2 cups green beans
- 2 cups diced celery
- 2 cups diced mushrooms
- 1 diced green peppers
- 3/4 cup diced onion
- 1/4 cup gluten-free vegetable stock

- 1 tbsp olive oil
- Salt and pepper
- 6 oz Boneless chicken breast

Instructions

1. Preheat oven to 350°F
2. Mix vegetables, vegetable stock, olive oil and pour into a casserole dish
3. Season chicken breast with olive oil, salt and pepper
4. Add it to the blend of vegetable and bake for 30 minutes
5. Serve hot

11. Mixed rice

Ingredients

- 1/3 cup gluten-free cooked rice
- 1 tsp cooking oil
- 1 cup chopped red onion
- 2 tbsp paprika
- 1 tbsp allspice mix
- Crushed cilantro
- Salt & pepper, to taste

Instructions

1. Sauté onions until translucent
2. Add paprika, allspice mix, salt and pepper
3. Drop in cooked rice and mix
4. Sprinkle crushed cilantro and serve

12. Tofu soup

Ingredients

- 3/4 cup diced onion
- 2 stalks diced celery
- 1 clove pressed garlic
- 3/4 cup gluten-free vegetable stock
- 1 diced red bell pepper
- 3 oz cubed tofu
- 1 tsp apple cider vinegar

Instructions

1. Sauté onions and garlic until translucent
2. Add bell pepper, celery, vegetable stock and bring to a boil for 10 minutes
3. Drop in tofu and simmer for 6 minutes
4. Season with salt, pepper, vinegar and serve with warm bread

13. Grilled chicken with vegetables

Ingredients

- 1/2 cup low-fat yogurt
- 1/2 tsp cumin powder
- 1/2 tsp coriander
- 1/2 tsp chopped red pepper
- 1/8 tsp ground allspice mix
- 1/2 tsp lemon juice
- 1 clove pressed garlic
- Salt - to taste

- 6 oz diced chicken breast
- 1 cup diced zucchini
- 1 cup diced summer squash
- 2 halved tomatoes

Instructions

- Preheat the grill.
- Blend spices with marinade ingredients
- Massage the blend onto chicken strips
- Sprinkle salt and pepper to taste
- Bake for 30 minutes and serve with toasted bread

14. Grilled chicken salad

Ingredients

- 3 oz cooked pre-cooked chicken breast
- 1 cup diced celery
- 3/4 cup diced red onion
- 2 tsp olive oil
- Allspice seasoning
- 1 tbsp chopped fresh mint
- 1 cup shredded romaine lettuce
- 1 cup shredded baby spinach

Instructions

1. In a salad bowl, mix chicken, celery, onion, oil, and mint
2. Toss olive oil to coat. Sprinkle with salt, pepper and allspice seasoning

3. Place a bed lettuce and spinach on a plate
4. Toss in the seasoned chicken and vegetables
5. Serve with bread sticks

Bonus Chapter

Let's face it, where there's good food, there's always room for a little MORE! Well, that's precisely why I've included a few more recipes to gorge on. I'd say it's time to feast on!

Bonus recipes for snacks, deserts and shakes

1. Couscous salad

Ingredients

- 175 g couscous
- 450 ml boiling water
- 200 g canned and drained tuna
- 50 g sliced sun-dried tomatoes
- 40 g black olives
- I onion finely chopped

For the dressing

- 3 tbsp olive oil
- 1 tbsp lemon juice
- 2-3 basil leaves
- Salt and pepper

Instructions

1. Pour boiling water over couscous in a bowl and set aside for 5 minutes
2. Add the remaining main ingredients along with the dressing ingredients and serve

2. Summer berry sundae

Ingredients

- 500 g assorted berries
- 3 tbsps blackcurrant cordial
- 250 g Greek yogurt
- 4 tbsp honey
- 2 tbsp chopped mint

Instructions

1. Blend the fruit and cordial until crushed and sorbet like
2. Add yogurt, honey and mint to the pureed mixture
3. Scoop into a wine glass and garnish with chopped mint leaves

3. Ginger-Berry Swirl

Ingredients

- 3 tablespoons of a protein powder of your choice
- 2 inch piece of peeled ginger
- 2 cups of dark leafy greens (could be any or a combination of kale, collards, romaine, spinach and/or chard)
- 1 cup of celery
- 1 cup assorted berries
- ½ cup water

Instructions

1. Blend all ingredients until smooth
2. Serve cold

Note: You can also include foods such as chia seeds, watermelon, and avocado and/or coconut water for variety.

Conclusion and Next Steps

I hope that by reading this book you have both- the answers to any questions you might have had on inflammation and the knowledge with which you can win the battle against it. Remember that controlling the symptoms of chronic inflammation while leading a happy and content life is possible, but you need to formulate a good plan (like the one I've provided in this e-book) and follow it consistently. You see, I share this book NOT because I want to seek attention from it, but because I know I have a formula that can do a lot of good to you. If you can follow the guidelines and recipes provided in this book with 100% intent, then I guarantee to deliver on its promise of reducing inflammation-related symptoms.

I've had a personally enriching experience writing this book and hope that it translates to you too. Remember that I am with you at every step of this journey and have your back at all times. Finally, if you liked this book, then make sure you read my other books too. I guarantee that you'll be equally pleased with the experience.

The Paleo Diet

The Paleo diet, similar to the anti-inflammation diet works at eliminating foods that are difficult to digest (grains, legumes and dairy) and including foods that increase the consumption of vitamins, minerals and antioxidants. Known to improve blood lipids, promote weight loss and reduce pain from intestinal problems, the diet delivers on its promise of promoting good health and reducing intestinal problems. Intrigued and keen to more? You can purchase my book by visiting: coming soon

Nutribullet Recipe Book

Here, I give you in-depth knowledge on the diet that's taken the fitness world by storm- The Nutribullet Diet. The diet emphasises on healthy living while showing you ways to incorporate liquid diets into your lifestyle. In my book, I share with you first-hand experiences and hand-picked recipes, its certain to leave you with the best detox plan you've ever known. Designed for detoxification, weight loss and healthy living, my book is sure to leave you inspired for live. You can purchase my book by visiting: coming soon

Bonus FREE Report – A gift from me to you

"6 Proven Health Benefits of Apple Cider Vinegar"

A miracle ingredient whose benefits range from healing skin allergies, killing harmful gut-bacteria, aiding digestion, controlling diabetes, reducing bad cholesterol, promoting weight loss, treating dandruff to preventing cancer and heart ailments, Apple Cider Vinegar is a versatile food component that goes beyond being just a cupboard-ingredient. In my book, I share with you the nutritional facts and beneficial properties of this highly handy fermented liquid. You can download my report by visiting: www.Freevinegar.com

Well, what are you waiting for? Make sure you grab a copy now!

Good luck!

Caroline

If you enjoyed this book can I please ask a favour, could you please leave me a review I would love to hear your feedback. It will only take a minute.

I thank you in advance

Made in the USA
Las Vegas, NV
22 November 2022

60056586R00039